RE

"Anyone reading this boo. .... by a 'cancer victor', whether you have cancer or not, can better understand how to triumph over adversity. How is it possible to say: 'Having cancer proved to be one of the most positive experiences of my life?' Don Denton experienced the answer, and shares lessons in this book that we all need to learn. His information on a powerful new cancer therapy is valuable; but more important is information on 'life therapy'. I recommend that anyone who fears hearing the 'C' word read this book immediately. It could change your life."

–Terry Douglass, CEO
Provision Healthcare, Knoxville, TN

Dr. Douglass is the driving force behind the development of the Provision Center for Proton Therapy in Knoxville. He is an exceptional Christ-follower and engineer, who has dedicated this world-class facility to Jesus Christ.

"Life's challenges are intimidating. In Calming the Storm Don Denton invites us on a journey of faith. Disappointment and discouragement are persistent adversaries. This book is a valuable tool for anyone walking through a season of shadows.

Faith in God opens doors of possibilities in many new ways. Don's candor about his journey extends hope for others. I recommend this book for anyone searching for a path through difficulties. It is a triumphant response to a life challenge."

–Allen Jackson, Senior Pastor

World Outreach Church, Murfreesboro, TN

Pastor Allen leads World Outreach Church of Murfreesboro, Tennessee, an incredible organization devoted to developing Christ-followers. My wife and I joined his tour to Israel in June 2013. While there, Allen challenged us to find the Holy Spirit's direction for our lives. This book is a direct response to His calling.

––––––––––––––

"When the word Cancer is mentioned in any doctor's office, fear, hopelessness and despair strike the very core of one's being. Don will show you that it doesn't have to be this way. This book is a must read for any individual looking for not only a physical cure but a spiritual one as well."

–J. P. Wilson, Senior Pastor

Liberty Church, Foley, AL

Pastor J. P. and his wife, Melissa, have hearts of gold in their efforts to enlarge the kingdom. He is leading the spiritual renewal of lower Alabama and having a positive impact on its communities.

"Mr Denton's story is one I have heard many times before. From a patient's perspective, he accurately describes the journey from diagnosis to treatment as a journey in faith, with milestones marked by Biblical references of encouragement and promise. It is a great testimony of encouragement."

–Dr. Nancy Mendenhall, Medical Director
University of Florida Proton Therapy Institute,
Jacksonville, FL

Dr. Mendenhall spearheaded the development of UFPTI, and she has been instrumental in promoting proton therapy as a cancer treatment option. She is recognized as one of the top cancer doctors in the world.

"A passage from the Bible seems to describe Don Denton's journey to healing from cancer: 'Dear friend, I pray that you may enjoy good health and that all may go well with you, even as your soul is getting along well.' I was privileged to have a front row seat to the spiritual growth he experienced during the weeks of treatments in Jacksonville. His positive

attitude and passion for a life worth living combined with groundbreaking treatment for a great story of success. I hope you enjoy his insights as I have."

–The Rt Rev., Dr. Daniel Williams

Ponte Vedra, FL

Daniel founded Christ the Redeemer Church in Ponte Vedra, Florida, which my wife and I attended during my cancer treatments. He served as my spiritual mentor during this time and always had the most profound and perfect words of encouragement to me.

Calming

THE

STORM

A CHRIST-FOLLOWER'S
VICTORY OVER CANCER

Calming
THE
STORM

A CHRIST-FOLLOWER'S
VICTORY OVER CANCER

DON DENTON

DEDICATION

I dedicate this book to my dad, Fred Denton, who succumbed in 1985 to his own battle with colon cancer when conventional treatment methods at the time didn't work. From diagnosis to death only six months passed, and he suffered greatly.

While dad never had much materially, he was the richest person spiritually that I've ever known. He was a true Christ-follower in every sense. I credit him for being the greatest positive influence in my life. God blessed me tremendously with the privilege of being his son.

The fantastic news is that his passing ushered in a new chapter in his existence–one that will last for eternity. He resides forever with the King of Kings, our Lord and Savior, our Redeemer, and our best friend, Jesus Christ. When your loved ones die, know that if given a choice of remaining in heaven or returning to earth, you should rejoice that you won't see them again until your time comes. Heaven is the reward for all believers who have the faith to accept God's wondrous gift of grace offered through Jesus Christ's ultimate sacrifice of Himself.

Dad taught me valuable lessons that still ring in my ears and benefit me today. During my career in the positions that I served with various companies, I enjoyed the privilege of working with many corporate business leaders in North America, the Far East, and Western

Europe. However, they weren't as successful as my dad. Unlike them, he didn't have possessions, education, money, power or status, but he was rich in the areas of life that really mean the most. He emulated Jesus Christ in remarkable ways.

He taught me these valuable life lessons:

–Serve others, and love them more than you love yourself;

–Realize that God owns everything, and you're merely a steward of what He has allowed you to handle during your time on earth;

–Give generously;

–Recognize everyone's value, as all are made in the image of God;

–Do good, and don't seek any recognition or thanks for doing so;

–Honesty is always the best policy; more importantly, it is the only policy;

–Live within your means, and address needs but not desires;

–Never give less than your best.

I could provide many examples of how he practiced what he taught with his own life, but that'd require a book of its own. Dad was a remarkable man, and more importantly, an outstanding role model as a Christian. I learned more applications of spiritual principles from him than from all the preachers, church teachers, and everyone else combined that I've known over the years.

Dad generously gave me the great legacy of his life. While it'd be admirable to say that I want to be just like him, the truth is that my goal—and hopefully yours—is to be more like Jesus.

To Fred Denton I dedicate this book. I pray that it will benefit you in conquering the cancer in your life, whether it's a physical disease or a spiritual disease.

TABLE OF CONTENTS

Foreword xi

Introduction 1

Blessings May Come from the Strangest
    of Places 3

The Little "c" 11

All Doctors Aren't Created Equal 17

Why Don? 25

Hope from Finding the Best Kept Secret
    in Medicine 37

The Amazing Transformation from Despair
    to Expectation 45

Florida or Bust 55

Favored 61

D-Day Finally Arrives 65

Jeremiah 29:11 71

Off to the Races 81

The New Normal 87

Bottom Line: What You Really Must Know 91

The New Paradigm for Curing Cancer 99

Closing 105

Acknowledgements 107

FOREWORD

In the weeks following the not-so-pleasant news: "You have cancer," my dad struggled with the question, "What now?" He didn't like what he heard about conventional treatment, and he desperately sought out more information from other men who had already trodden this road. A chance conversation led him to proton therapy, then a little-known option that no one else had mentioned by name.

Maybe you are seeking out more information, or maybe you are looking for that person who has been there before to open up and describe his experiences—without hesitation or embarrassment. This book is that conversation: one man's honest account of his thoughts and fears on diagnosis, the process of his treatment, and his results in life after cancer.

My dad simply wants anyone who can benefit from proton therapy to know about it. This is his story.

–Brian Denton

I, for one, am very privileged to know the author of this book on a very personal level. He's my dad. I grew up knowing him my entire life. I witnessed a lot of his ups and downs; I learned many life lessons from him; I know his interests and what he loves. To me, Don Denton is more than just a dad—he's a mentor and a very dear friend. That's why learning that he was diagnosed with cancer was devastating.

Cancer. It's a very frightening word, especially when you or someone you love suffers from it. To most, cancer means you're doomed. However, Dad (and our entire family) was very blessed when he discovered the hidden gem of medical science: proton therapy.

This book entails my dad's trials and tribulations, his struggles, and ultimately his victory over cancer. I wish that readers of this book are ignited with a spark of hope that cancer *can* be beaten.

–Andrew Denton

FRONT COVER CREDIT

On this body of water, Jesus Christ performed the miracle of calming the storm. An account appears in Luke 8:22-25 (NIV):

22 One day Jesus said to his disciples, "Let us go over to the other side of the lake." So they got into a boat and set out.

23 As they sailed, he fell asleep. A squall came down on the lake, so that the boat was being swamped, and they were in great danger.

24 The disciples went and woke him, saying, "Master, Master, we're going to drown!"

He got up and rebuked the wind and the raging waters; the storm subsided, and all was calm.

25 "Where is your faith?" he asked his disciples.

In fear and amazement they asked one another, "Who is this? He commands even the winds and the water, and they obey him."

INTRODUCTION

This book has been written primarily for anyone who has been diagnosed with cancer and is trying to figure out what to do. Secondarily it's for the people who love and care about you. I empathize with your dilemma, because I've been there myself. It's not easy sorting through all the information and making life-affecting decisions on your own.

Having cancer is a battle: emotionally, physically, and spiritually. It will change you. In my experience, I not only survived but thrived, and became a better person because of it. I want the same for you.

At this stage you're likely buried in trying to learn as much as you can. It takes a lot of time to sort out everything you come across. For this reason, I've deliberately cut to the chase in writing a book about my personal journey that can be read quickly in one to two hours.

I believe that it will give you valuable insights that you are unlikely to learn anywhere else. It is brutally honest and revealing. While everyone's situation is a little different, you'll likely see some similarities in your journey as compared to mine.

God bless you in the days ahead. Keep the faith! Never give up! You, too, can be victorious over cancer.

Chapter One

BLESSINGS MAY COME FROM THE STRANGEST OF PLACES

FOR YEARS I HAVE STRUGGLED on-and-off with high blood pressure and slightly elevated cholesterol. Multiple doctors have attempted to help me, but to no avail in terms of a long-term solution. With a few pills, the blood pressure would come down, and with better diet, the cholesterol would improve, only to head right back up in a few months.

It's a condition that has annoyed me for over thirty years. I've remained steadfastly mindful of the potential health risks, since my dad experienced two heart attacks during his lifetime, and Susie, my wife and into healthy living, suffered a widower-maker heart attack in 2006 at the young age of 53. (By the way, she survived when the odds were squarely against her, due to a miraculous intervention of God.)

We lived in Bowling Green, Kentucky, for 26 years. For five of the last six years we were there, I maintained a business office 83 miles away in Franklin, Tennessee, south of Nashville. The daily three-hour roundtrip commute proved grueling. One day while driving home in rush hour traffic, my left arm started *misbehaving*. My mind quickly ascertained that maybe, just maybe, a heart attack was imminent. I detoured and drove to Vanderbilt Medical Center Emergency. After many hours of extensive questioning and testing, the doctor released me with a diagnosis of having no idea of what caused my problem, along with a bill of several thousand dollars for his analysis. Thank goodness that I had great health insurance at the time. After he exited the examining room, a gracious nurse stopped by before I was released. She said to me, "I'm not supposed to tell you this, because I'm not a doctor. Don't let him know that I've spoken with you. I've seen your type of case several times. You're a prime candidate for a stroke. Watch out and be careful. When you return to Bowling Green, I suggest seeing your regular doctor and discussing what happened with him."

As it turned out, in the short-term things settled down for me until my wife's heart attack. Her experience triggered a total change in our lifestyle. I decided to leave the corporate rat race with its ceaseless demands, incredible work hours, and overall stress of being a high-ranking officer over the previous 26 years. While the fruits of my employment had blessed us tremendously, it had also taken a toll on both my and Susie's health. Given a choice between continuing the grind or protecting our health, choosing health was a no-brainer. I threw in the towel, and happily acknowledged that the rats had won!

When Susie and I became engaged in 1972, we shared our hopes and dreams of the future–just as all couples typically do. In this important setting of getting to know each other better, we learned that we possessed a common desire: to have two homes–one in the mountains and one on the coast. (I readily admit our thinking contradicted my dad's guidance of fulfilling needs but not desires.) People who know us well understand that we're long-term planners and executers. Today we have both, and despite what some people may think, luck had absolutely nothing to do with it. God had everything to do with it, and we are merely stewards of what he has entrusted to us during our days on earth.

Within 16 months of Susie's near-death, we moved from Bowling Green into our beautiful new mountain home in East Tennessee. Our property is nestled against the Great Smoky Mountains National Park in as peaceful a location that one could ever have. Even though I decided to be a consulting engineer on a very limited basis of a few hours monthly, I really had no stress. Life was very good.

However, nothing changed relative to my high blood pressure, but with medication my cholesterol level gradually dropped over time. Our regular family doctor started trying different medicines to address this issue, along with a recommendation to lose 30 pounds. I bought a good cuff monitor and checked my blood pressure daily at roughly the same time.

Every single month, I met with my doctor to review the results. He continually changed my medicine, trying one thing and then another, and tweaking the dosage up and down. I hate popping pills, because the potential side effects are worse than the ailment. Nothing seemed to work with any reliability, as my blood pressure measurements were all over the map—sometimes too high and sometimes too low.

One evening I was preparing to take a shower, and I passed out. Our master bathroom has plenty of hard surfaces to crack one's skull or break some bones. When I went down, I simply crumpled and didn't hit anything that hurt me. In retrospect, it was simply amazing. In a short while I could hear my wife asking rather silly questions (like what's your name; who's your doctor, etc.), and I attempted to answer her. Rather than wait an indefinite time for an ambulance to arrive from 20 miles away, she placed me in the car and we took off to the University of Tennessee Medical Center. The experience proved similar to what had happened a couple of years earlier at Vanderbilt. They questioned and tested me at length. However, unlike the Vanderbilt doctor who had no opinion on what had happened to me, the Tennessee doctor determined that I had fainted! Again, the bill was thousands of dollars and I was grateful to have good health insurance.

I returned to my regular doctor, who ordered more tests. He decided to start doing blood work every month to monitor any changes. In this connection, he checked my PSA, which is an initialism for *protein specific antigen*. I never gave it a second thought, because it was just one of a laundry list of blood characteristics that he checked.

A few weeks later, on a Sunday afternoon at nearby gift shop, I started feeling badly–very badly. I located my wife and she drove us home. I immediately checked my blood pressure and found it to be 200 over 110. We jumped into the car and headed to the University of Tennessee Medical Center once again. The doctor gave me an IV with medicine to reduce my blood pressure to a safe level, and sent me home.

Fortunately, this event has (so far!) marked my last trip to a hospital for blood pressure problems. However, I continued to see my regular doctor on a monthly basis, and he continued to play around with various medications to find a combination that would work. This process went on for month after month after month. I eventually lost patience and felt like my issue would never be resolved. After these experiences with many doctors I started questioning in my own mind how smart these guys really are. You'll find out soon how this realization helped me tremendously.

Every month when I'd meet my doctor, he'd review the daily blood pressure readings that I'd taken and the blood work results that the lab had determined. Eventually he started noting my PSA and the PSA velocity, the rate at which it was increasing. He opined that odds were 50/50 that nothing was wrong, but he recommended that I see a urologist for further analysis.

My regular doctor set up an appointment for me to visit a urologist in a nearby practice, reputedly the best one in the greater Knoxville area. A few days later I found myself filling out forms, having my insurance checked, and going in to see him. After looking over my medical history and asking a few questions, he did a DRE, which sounds a lot better than *Digital Rectal Exam*. As a man gets older, his prostate may gradually enlarge and become harder. A skilled doctor can determine by feel the possibility of something being wrong. In my case, he found my prostate to be a proper size and texture, which suggests, but certainly doesn't assure, that one doesn't have prostate cancer. However, I had this little issue of an escalating PSA, which measured 4.6 at the time but had also increased by a full point over the past six months. My appointment ended with him telling me that he wanted to do a biopsy, so I set up a return visit for a couple of weeks later.

If you haven't had this procedure, just know that it's not a lot of fun. I regard myself as one with a high pain threshold. If caught by the enemy, I wouldn't reveal any more than my name, rank, and serial number, even under torture.

The urologist took twelve plugs out of my prostate and plotted the location of each one. The basic idea is to sample tissue from throughout the gland and check for cancer cells.

Quite frankly, I'm glad he had removed the front sight from the 22 that he inserted in my behind, because the 12 shots he fired hurt enough on their own.

Everything from my biopsy was neatly packaged and sent to a pathologist in nearby Oak Ridge who specializes in examining cells with an electron microscope and rendering an opinion. I had to wait anxiously for days before receiving a response.

Cast your cares on the Lord and he will sustain you;
he will never let the righteous fail.
–PSALM 55:22

Chapter Two

THE LITTLE "C"

MY CELL PHONE RANG just after the Cracker Barrel server had delivered our lunch to us on a gorgeous October day in 2010. As I pulled it out of my pocket, the urologist's number showed up, so I took the call.

"Don, this is 'Jane' (fictitious name) and I'm calling for Dr. 'Smith' (another fictitious name). You have cancer. Can you stop by the office this afternoon so we can talk?" How do you answer such a question except with a weak "yes" that is barely audible as it gets out of your mouth? Our conversation ceased as quickly as it had started and I hung up the phone.

Wow! The bluntness of the urologist's assistant stunned me almost as much as her news. She must not have taken People Skills 101. Her words impacted me with the force of an atom bomb. Delivering bad news requires a lot more finesse to ease the person into being able to receive it. However, my reaction was influenced more by the message than the messenger.

As a Christian, I recognize that everyone has their own faults and weaknesses, including myself. She may have been having a bad day or under some personal stress or just unaware of her presentation style. It really doesn't matter. My attitude is that no one can harm me with words; it's only how I respond to them that counts. I don't let myself be controlled by the circumstances. In this case, simply focusing on her news instead of her delivery proved to be the right course.

(As a follow-up, since our initial encounter, I have come to know "Jane" as a good friend. She is an exceptional and caring Christian lady, who does an absolutely remarkable job in helping others. She is truly concerned about patients and people who are hurting, as evidenced by her tireless efforts in many areas. A lot of folks are blessed as a result of having her in their lives.)

A message like that really ruins a lunch. It stunned me for learning the news that I really didn't expect to hear. I don't know why, but with the way I felt physically and my relatively young age of 62 years, I couldn't imagine that I was actually sick. After all, I had no symptoms whatsoever—at least not that I could sense.

Of course, my loving wife wanted the news, so I told her. She stopped eating. For the next few minutes, both of us had difficult moments of holding back tears. We had no idea what the news really meant or what the future held in store for us.

This particular lunch was the worse one ever at a Cracker Barrel, but it certainly had nothing to do with the restaurant. We scooted our food around on our plates and took occasional bites until we decided that we had enough.

The cheery cashier took my credit card and gleefully asked how I enjoyed my lunch. I took the easy way out and simply stated that it was fine. She smilingly promoted some candy but I quickly declined. I'm sure some people would have lit into her for no other reason than being at the wrong place at the wrong time. There's no way that I expected her to be sympathetic to my plight.

We drove less than 10 minutes from Cracker Barrel to reach the urologist's office, innocently located among hotels and restaurants. After signing in with the receptionist, we waited for an unseemly long time in the lobby for our turn. As I looked around to see who else was there, I noticed nothing but long faces of elderly patients. Apparently I had joined their ranks, but I certainly didn't feel deserving of membership in this not very exclusive club.

Finally my name was called by the frank assistant who had informed me that I have cancer, and she took us into a little room to talk.

She started by saying "You have cancer with a little 'c'. You don't have the big 'C'. You will make it through this trial just fine, and you'll be okay. You're not going to die. Just don't worry." My immediate internalized response was "That's easy for you to say, because you don't have a prostate and have no concept of what I will experience and feel as a man."

She moved on to the next part of her programmed pitch–one that I'm sure she has repeated a thousand times–by giving me an information packet about prostate cancer and the practice's allegedly fabulous medical team. It contained a book and some brochures. She instructed us to wait for a few minutes for the urologist to meet us.

Naturally, it took a long time before the doctor ever graced us with his presence. I suspect many of these guys are deliberately late to appointments to create an impression that they are incredibly busy professionals, occupied with the important task of saving lives. After all, compared to me at the time, he was clearly in the driver's seat and not scared.

He finally entered the room to meet with us, carrying a manila folder with my short medical history at his practice. My mind raced with dozens of thoughts and questions, since I knew nothing about my disease or the treatment options. I couldn't wait to hear his spiel and ask a few questions about my cancer with a little "c".

So do not fear, for I am with you;
do not be dismayed, for I am your God.

—Isaiah 41:10

Chapter Three

ALL DOCTORS ARE NOT CREATED EQUAL

AFTER A STONY INTRODUCTION, he started revealing what the biopsy showed. His style was matter-of-fact, direct, and authoritative, and as an engineer, that approach suited me just fine. Fortunately, in my dad's last days before he died from cancer, I had met his doctor on numerous occasions, so those experiences prepared me for this discussion on my own health. The dialogue sounded eerily familiar.

In a monotone voice in methodical fashion he said, "The pathologist's report shows that you have cancer with a Gleason score of 7. It's measured on a 2 to 10 scale, with 10 being the most aggressive. Your biopsy showed cancer in two samples. One is a 3 and one is a 4. So, 3 plus 4 equal 7."

I asked if it'd be advisable to have another pathologist examine the slides of the plugs out of my prostate gland to see if another opinion would emerge. He showed color photographs of the cells to me and explained that the only other possible conclusion would be that my Gleason score is actually a 6 or 8–either way, the fact that I had cancer was irrefutable and inescapable. I agreed with his logic.

He went on to say, "A 7 Gleason is a high medium in terms of aggressiveness. You don't have to address it immediately, but you should decide what to do within a month." My first impression was that "immediately" and "month" are synonyms.

His conversation took a dark tone as he continued, but I remained stoic during the process. I know my supportive wife sat directly next to me, but my attention focused squarely on the doctor and what he had to say.

The urologist started the process of educating me on the various treatment options. The good news about prostate cancer is that several techniques exist to address it; the bad news is that most of them aren't very good.

The short (paraphrased) version of his pitch went something like this: "My specialty is prostatectomy using state-of-the-art da Vinci robotic equipment, and this option fits your situation very well. It is the gold standard for treating prostate cancer. I do surgery twice weekly, preferably at Ft. Sanders but also at

Blount Memorial. The whole process would take about four hours, including anesthesia, the operation, etc. You'd remain in the hospital overnight and likely go home the next day. You'd wake-up from surgery with a catheter in your urethra in order to urinate. It will remain intact for a few days, depending on how well you recover. Following my directions, you should be up and about soon thereafter and recover completely within 6 months."

"What is the probability of successfully eliminating my cancer and the related side effects?", I asked. His blunt reply blindsided me completely: "With surgery, you have a 65% likelihood of living for 10 years with no recurrence; you'll be permanently incontinent and impotent. After this timeframe the probability of recurrence is fairly high." I followed with "How many of these have you done?", which he answered with the non-answer of *lots*, as if I had insulted him for questioning his experience level.

I guess that I should have been thankful for his assistant's assurance that I had cancer with a little "c" instead of the big "C", but thankfulness isn't the first thought that entered my mind. Quite frankly, I'd rather be dead than to be permanently incontinent and impotent and not knowing if my cancer were making a comeback. The big "C" seemed strangely more palatable than the little "c". Have it, suffer greatly for a short while, then die and proceed to heaven, sort of like a *Get*

Out of Jail Free card in Monopoly. It didn't sound too bad. Conversely, the little "c" with huge quality of life issues and uncertainty seemed more like the Chinese torture of *death by a thousand cuts*, the process whereby small plugs of flesh are taken from a person's body with the objective that he'd die slowly but surely after a long duration of agonizing pain and suffering. I surely didn't want *that*, but *that* is what the doctor offered, and he called it the *Gold Standard*. It sounded more like the tin standard to me. I could hardly wait to hear how bad the other options are.

He went on to tell me his second recommendation, brachytherapy. It's a technique in which the prostate is packed with radioactive seeds to stop the cancer growth by destroying the cells' DNA to prevent it from reproducing. It could be done in one day at the hospital. My urologist would not actually insert the seeds, but he'd be there to assist the radiologist as necessary. He opined that the outcome would be about the same as the prostatectomy—in other words, horrible.

The third option has a really innocent sounding name, watchful waiting. Quite frankly, it appealed to me. It involved no surgery, no pain, no hospital time, etc. You just be careful with your lifestyle relative to eating and exercising, and take a PSA test every three months to see what happens. It also sounds really dumb for someone of my age. *Watchful waiting*—what are you waiting for? It's the ultimate procrastinator's choice for dealing with cancer. Granted, if you're up in years, it would make some sense. To the urologist's credit, he didn't recommend it.

High Intensity Focused Ultrasound (HIFU) came in as option four. This method concentrates high frequency sound waves on the cancerous tissue, heating it up and killing the cells. The urologist stated that it wasn't legal in this country at the time, but he offered to direct me to the right place in some third-world country. Can you believe that he even mentioned this one?

Number five didn't come across as a real option. The urologist simply said, "Some guys go to Jacksonville, but it takes two months and who'd want to do that?" He didn't elaborate whatsoever, and I didn't ask because my mind had continued to process the information dump that he had just provided.

Just paint me naive, as something very clearly orchestrated had gradually unfolded in the urologist's presentation, but I didn't recognize it at the time. His recommendations corresponded exactly to what he does to earn a living. He'd make the most money doing a robotic prostatectomy (option one) and less money assisting the radiologist with the brachytherapy (option two). He didn't recommend any treatment option that would deprive him from making a buck.

At this point he went for the hard sell. "Looking at your biopsy and DRE results, I think your cancer has metastasized—that is, spread beyond your prostate. It's likely that you'll have to have surgery followed by radiation and hormone shots," he confidently asserted. Be mindful of this one simple fact: he made this statement without doing any tests whatsoever to back it up. In retrospect, it wasn't just intelligent analysis based upon specialized education and years of experience, but a rehearsed pitch to scare the you-know-what out of me.

To his great credit, he instructed me to *do my homework* and pick the right option for me. As you'll learn later, I embraced his suggestion wholeheartedly. It proved to be the best advice that he gave to me.

I closed by asking him what he would do if he were I. With no hesitation, he said the robotic prostatectomy, but he assured me that I had to make the decision. Silly me, I thought the doctor should tell me what to do rather than just lay out the options for me to pick one. After all, isn't it one of the reasons why he makes the big bucks?

His closing statement was priceless after unloading all his earlier information and opinions. He said, "Take some time to evaluate what I've told you. However, with your cancer spreading, you can't afford to wait. You must make a decision within a month, but I suggest three weeks. In the meantime, I'll look at my schedule and let you know when you could have surgery."

I thanked him for his time, and left the office slightly more informed but greatly more perplexed. In spite of being diagnosed with cancer and not knowing what awaited me in the weeks ahead, and in a state of disillusionment and despair, I clearly realized that I have a loving God who cares for me and would get me through this ordeal intact. Since He even knows the number of hairs on my head, curing me would be absolutely no issue for Him. I had the great opportunity to prove that faith works.

That evening I reflected on the day's events, and a feeling of tremendous thankfulness came over me. You see, I never knew that I had cancer, because I had not experienced any of the indicators. I felt perfectly fine and in good health. Only because I had a blood pressure problem did I come to be diagnosed with cancer. If it had not taken so long to solve this totally unrelated issue, which drove the need for more and more blood tests, I would have remained dumb and happy and never realized the severity of my greater health problem.

In previous months I had become impatient and disappointed by my regular doctor's inability to reduce and stabilize my blood pressure, but at the end of the day, his failure proved to be a tremendous success. Knowing that I had cancer and merely having to figure out how to defeat it proved to be more comforting than remaining ignorant and passive.

Blessings may come from the strangest places. It certainly occurred in my case.

For the revelation awaits an appointed time; it speaks of the end and will not prove false. Though it linger, wait for it; it will certainly come and will not delay.

—HABAKKUK 2:3

Chapter Four

WHY DON?

Upon leaving the urologist's office I headed straight for a bookstore to see what it might have relative to prostate cancer. After looking through the skimpy offerings, I picked out two books to read. Combined with the information packet provided by the urologist's assistant, I had plenty of material to pour over the rest of the day.

For the next several hours I devoured everything that I had accumulated. Education is a great thing. My theory is that the more you learn, the dumber you get, because you ultimately realize that there's so much more to know than you ever imagined initially.

I checked out all the treatment options that the urologist had told me: robotic surgery, radiation seeds, doing nothing, and ultrasound heating–everything except the mysterious and undefined option in Jacksonville, since he gave me no clue as to what it is.

Being an engineer can be a blessing and a curse. On the plus side, we're analytical and methodical in gathering facts and solving problems. On the minus side, we want to know the minutiae, which may result in procrastination in reaching a decision. Our lofty but usually unattainable goal is perfection.

We tend to see things in black and white, whereas the real world is generally gray. All you engineers and spouses know exactly what I mean. Unfortunately, the medical world falls squarely into the gray category, which is exasperating to us techies.

The right side of my brain kicked in, so I followed the usual route with step number one: listing the pros and cons of every treatment option. Every engineer knows the next step. After making a nice table of this information, I assigned a point value of importance to each characteristic. After tallying the totals by treatment option, the best one for me should clearly emerge. It makes perfect sense, right?

I could not have been more wrong. The real difficulty is that this exercise showed every option to be pretty lousy. It's impossible to choose one just after ranking all of them with cumulative low scores. It's like being on death row and having to pick hanging, injection or electrocution. However, in the case of prostate cancer, it's akin to selecting the type of long-term torture that you prefer.

Many resources exist to inform one about the positives and negatives of treatment options, so I won't elaborate on them. However, just to give you a flavor of the decision-making process, I'll share some basics of what I learned very early in my analysis.

First, robotic surgery is oftentimes accompanied by impotence and incontinence. The surgeon usually doesn't remove the entire prostate, so tissue is left over that may still be cancerous or he/she may spread the cancer while removing pieces of the gland. Also, the urethra passes right through it, so upon removal a man's penis is usually shortened by an inch or so as well. Recovery for many men is slow. Both temporary and permanent side effects are part of the course. This procedure certainly sounds like the Gold Standard! It must be great, because my urologist ranked robotic surgery his #1 recommendation!

Second, radioactive seeds—usually several hundred of them—are packed into the prostate through an incision in one's bottom. The radiation given off damages the DNA of the cells and prevents them from dividing and reproducing. If an errant seed is deposited into a man's urethra, problems such as permanent incontinence may occur. In past times, the seeds could drift and wind up in parts of the body where they certainly don't belong and cause issues. However, nowadays I understand that most are strung together to prevent drifting.

Third, watchful waiting is a choice made by many men after they learn about robotic surgery and radioactive seeds. It reflects wishful thinking and a desire to die of some other cause before the prostate cancer takes them out. Quite frankly, this option registered pretty high with me at the end of the day. The others seemed fraught with so many problems that I'd rather do nothing other than hope and pray. To my urologist's credit, he spoke against watchful waiting. However, I suspect his opinion was biased by how much money he'd make if I selected one of his recommended options.

Fourth, High Intensity Focused Ultrasound (HIFU) didn't even register with me after the urologist explained that I'd have to do it in some third world country if I decided to make this choice. I don't know anything about it and never seriously considered it after hearing the word "illegal". I figured that the particular technique must be fraught with problems since it couldn't be performed here.

Fifth, I had no clue what going to Jacksonville for two months even meant. None of the materials provided by the urologist's office or picked up at the bookstore provided any hint of what this choice is all about. In the ensuing days I didn't become any more informed.

In a nutshell, my options after some analysis appeared to be robotic surgery, radiation seeds, and watchful waiting. On the plus side, my total absorption of as much information as possible kept my mind too busy to feel sorry for myself.

Expanding my knowledge base occupied me totally for the next several days. I went to another bookstore and bought additional books on prostate cancer, stopped by the county library and checked out books, and spent endless hours on the internet absorbing information like a sponge. Also, I started networking by talking with other men who had previously traveled this path. Some were relatives, friends, and business associates, but most were referrals. Cancer has a way of coalescing survivors. Everyone who I contacted spoke with me patiently and kindly, and their level of support and concern was encouraging. However, as I learned later but not at this time, many men who have experienced prostate cancer don't open up (as they should) out of fear and embarrassment about the difficulties they have faced post-treatment.

Everything that I learned merely increased my education on the options presented by my urologist. After many hours of research, the same information came up time and again. It became so repetitive, and my learning curve eventually flattened out as nothing new was gleaned.

One of the life lessons I've instilled into my own sons is to evaluate the upside and downside in every situation. Using this same process to look at robotic surgery and radiation seeds only made them illogical choices undeserving of my selection. Learning more only pushed me closer to watchful waiting.

For an engineer, the process is maddening. We pursue the perfect solution to every problem, and so far the best that I could muster to address my own problem was to *do nothing*. Intuitively, this choice seemed very wrong. What a dilemma!

I knew the urologist had recommended surgery, and he wanted to do it in very early January. In retrospect I realize his recommendation resulted from this procedure being his specialty and the one whereby he'd earn the most money. When I had last spoken with him in his office, he seemed a little put out that I actually questioned him about other options and asked for further time to evaluate all of them.

After many days of an exhaustive effort of studying a new subject that possessed an incredible and seemingly uncontrollable dominance over me, I became depressed, worried, and a little agitated at even the little things. I started imagining my love life coming to a quick and abrupt end. Even a trip to the grocery almost made me cry upon seeing the shelf space dedicated to adult diapers. I thought that I might be buying them soon for my own use. *Impotence* and *incontinence* are two words no male wants to hear. They possess the crushing ability to make him feel like he's not a man. I had rather be dead—another plus for *watchful waiting*. At least I could die a man.

Unbeknown to me, during this same timeframe my dear wife, Susie, faced her own spiritual battle inside, blaming God for my cancer. I guess that's par for the course for us less-than-perfect humans. She became upset at Him for causing my disease. That's what she really felt. Be mindful that she's incredibly spiritual: a Christ-follower, Bible reader, prayer warrior—the whole nine yards. And, her faith was shaken to its very core. She couldn't imagine her life as a widow or as married to a depressed soul who no longer cared to live.

Susie remained quiet in her thoughts, and never shared them with me at the time. I suppose that she didn't want to alarm or upset me, and that she felt a need to be the strong right arm on which I could lean.

Nonetheless, her constant thought was "Why Don?" as she questioned God. She didn't ask it as a rhetorical question. She wanted an answer. I'm not sure a voice from the heavens or a burning bush or writing on stone tablets would have satisfied her. I had cancer that would either disable or kill me, and it was God's fault.

I don't criticize her reasoning. It showed her humanness. Even though I'm a Christ-follower, my natural tendency (as a result of my inherent sin-nature) is to forget about God when things are rolling along just fine and to become a mighty prayer warrior when things turn badly. I suspect most Christians act the same way.

Cancer is a big deal. It moves into a totally different level of seriousness when it's not someone else, but the guy looking back at you in the mirror.

Unlike my wife, I didn't blame God. Sometimes I think that technical people have a greater difficulty relating on an emotional and spiritual level, because they're so stinking rational and logical. It may be a difficult concept to explain, but blind faith to a techie still involves a high level of analysis; however, when they're *in*, they're *all in*. They typically aren't lukewarm Christians.

Consequently, I viewed my cancer as a biological event that just happened to me. My dad had died from colon cancer and he may have had prostate cancer but didn't know it. I regarded my misfortune as likely a genetic issue. I guess that I could have rationalized that God gave it to me since He wired my DNA, but I just didn't think this way. I wasn't the first and wouldn't be the last person faced with the tough decision on how to treat cancer.

Susie's primary support system is her family. She's one of eighteen kids–nine boys and nine girls. Their ages span a long time. As you can imagine, her siblings show tremendous differences in behavior, thinking, speaking, and relating. While one can see a family resemblance among them, their personalities vary all over the map and have diverged even more over time. My wife is the single most unique member of her family. She possesses traits molded by years of experiences and spiritual growth that distinguish her as an individual. She is an incredible woman.

My wife chatted primarily with her sisters about the battle we faced together. Interestingly, although she is closer to her younger sisters near her own age, it turned out that an older sister proved to be the one who awakened her to reality. This dear lady is always clear and direct with her opinions. One doesn't have to guess how she feels about anything.

Susie called her one day just to have a sympathetic soul to listen to her. She opined that I'm a great husband and father, and it seemed so unfair that I had been diagnosed with cancer when bad people in the world seemingly don't have such issues but richly deserve them. She couldn't understand why God would permit such a travesty to happen. In conclusion she asked THE question, "Why Don?"

Her sister responded immediately and authoritatively, "Why NOT Don?" To all the empty days and restless nights that my wife had agonized over this situation, a simple three-word answer snapped her mind and spirit back to reality.

Susie reflected on her sister's very direct response and knew absolutely, positively, unequivocally, beyond any shadow-of-doubt that it was right. Isn't it wonderful how God uses people? Who would have ever guessed that the u-turn in my wife's thinking would occur in this way? This simple event shows that we can learn from absolutely everyone. No one has all the answers and insights, but someone out there—someone you may not expect whatsoever—may have exactly what you need.

My wife changed her focus. She realized that God didn't give me cancer. This disease, like many others, is particularly insidious. Most psychologists believe that prostate cancer damages a man's psyche more than any other, as it robs him of his manhood before it takes his life. It's the ultimate kicking you while you're down, only in this case we're talking about life and death.

Her mindset transitioned quickly into *Satan caused Don's cancer.* In retrospect, it became easy for her to realize this very real conclusion. I suspect that she asked God for forgiveness in doubting His incomprehensible and inexhaustible love for us. Now, equipped with the right focus, she dedicated herself to praising and thanking God for the miracle that she fully expected Him to perform in my life using the instruments that He would choose to heal me and restore my health completely.

This experience changed everything. Both of us were in overdrive to find God's solution for my life. We didn't know how or when, but we had zero doubt that it would happen perfectly as He worked in our lives.

It didn't take long. Soon God orchestrated the encounters that literally transformed my life.

He causes his sun to rise on the evil and the good, and sends rain on the righteous and the unrighteous.

–Matthew 5:45b

Chapter Five

HOPE FROM FINDING THE BEST-KEPT SECRET IN MEDICINE

My phone rang and I received an unexpected call from my urologist's assistant, the one who had abruptly informed me of my positive cancer diagnosis. She invited my wife and me to a Christmas dinner with the local prostate cancer support group that would be held in a few days just a couple of miles from our home. She let me know that attendance would be high, and there would be men there who had experienced all the available treatment options, and I might learn something from talking with them. On the plus side, I thought it'd be great to meet more of these guys face-to-face and see their eyes when I asked tough questions. On the minus side, I felt the information gleaned would reinforce all the negative stuff that I already knew.

When the day arrived, I really didn't care to go. However, something inside of both my wife and me said to do so. In retrospect I know that nudge came from the Holy Spirit. He is reliable and dependable. We prepared some covered dishes of delicious food and assumed a more positive attitude of expectancy that something good would be learned.

When we arrived at the dinner, a lot of people were already there. Old couples, husbands and wives, carrying their covered dishes for everyone to enjoy. I felt so out-of-place. I didn't belong there. I was much too young and physically able to be in the same category as these guys.

Realizing that these folks would eat and run–a characteristic behavior of this age group–my wife and I knew immediately that we had to network with as many as possible to learn whatever we could. We were primed and ready to roll with predetermined questions to educate ourselves as much as possible.

As a couple we approached our first couple and after a brief introduction, fired away with questions. The husband had selected robotic surgery as his treatment option a couple of years earlier. He excitedly reported a positive experience with no problems whatsoever. In fact, he claimed that his sexual prowess had improved as a result of the surgery! Everything worked a-ok and could not be any better! His reply caught us totally off-guard as we didn't expect to hear anything like it. After a little more chit-chat, we broke away to talk between ourselves.

Compared to everything we had learned leading up to this conversation, his claims didn't make any sense. My smart-thinking wife opined that with her presence next to me, I wouldn't receive any truthful answers, as men wouldn't want to admit that they had issues in front of a new woman that they had just met. So, we took a divide and conquer approach in reassuming our recon roles. We'd separate a couple via casual conversation and quiz them independently about their experiences.

This tactic worked brilliantly. At least it turned out well for learning the truth from half the couples–the wives. My conversations with several husbands–those who had been treated with every option and who could teach me much–failed to provide forthright information. They wouldn't acknowledge any issues, even when confronted with my very pointed questions. Thankfully, their wives came through. In talking with my wife, they expressed great sadness at what their husbands had become. The men in their lives had serious quality of life issues. Many had sexual difficulties as a result of being made impotent by their treatment. Several had to wear adult diapers, as they had been made incontinent by their treatment. The stories matched exactly what I had learned over the previous weeks of research.

After talking with a half-dozen couples, our attention was diverted to eating dinner. We continued to work the table where we were seated, with Susie speaking with the women and me speaking with the men, although our physical closeness made the task difficult. Again and again, we heard the same kinds of reports.

At this one setting, they had the opportunity, the responsibility—yes, the moral obligation—to tell me like it is. Yet, they failed, every single one we had met up to that point. Nonetheless, I understand their feelings and why they didn't share their true stories with me. They were embarrassed and their pride wouldn't allow them to disclose their problems. They simply didn't want to talk about them. In this sense, they were deceptive, but I'm certain that they had no malice. However, had I followed their advice, I would be dead or wishing I were dead today. Fortunately, and I thank God for her, my wife dug down deep and obtained the truth from their wives. Problems abounded and lives were shattered; but the conventional treatments beat death, and that's the primary good that could be said about them.

Nonetheless, apart from this negative, the social aspect of the Christmas luncheon proved enjoyable. Reports of events past and future were given, photos were taken, new calendars were passed out, and everyone received some kind of small gift—mainly advertising trinkets promoting some drug-maker's product. We received a large canvas bag to use on the beach, marked with giant letters spelling *Cialis*. Now that's something every man would really like to use and announce to the world!

At this juncture the event began to dismantle as everyone started picking up and cleaning up to head home. Susie and I had spoken with only a few couples, but the tales we had heard didn't excite us about talking with any more. I felt downcast as the experience had only served to reinforce my greatest apprehensions about selecting a treatment for which the cure would be worse than the disease. My naive optimism had not been rewarded, but hope suddenly appeared on the horizon.

The next introduction literally changed my life—our lives. Two gentlemen and their wives approached us and introduced themselves. I had met one of the men on a couple of occasions previously, but didn't really know him.

All four people bombarded us with their personal stories of the husbands being cured of prostate cancer through a little-known treatment method known as proton therapy. We didn't have to separate them as we did the other couples, because they were singing off of the same sheet of sweet music. They literally talked over each other and were absolutely effervescent on how wonderful the experience had been for them. They executed an information dump faster than my mind could process it, and I scarcely had the chance to take it all in or ask a question.

The husbands explained that they had no surgery, no side effects, and no quality of life issues whatsoever. The wives talked about having a *radiation vacation* during their 8-9 weeks in Jacksonville.

Bingo! We heard the word *Jacksonville!* Proton therapy turned out to be the mysterious treatment that my urologist had said, "Some guys go to Jacksonville, but it takes two months and who'd want to do that?" Well, from the high praises of our newest and dearest friends, it certainly merited some serious evaluation.

Quite frankly, we found it difficult to believe them. After a few weeks of extensive research on conventional treatment options for prostate cancer, this proton therapy sounded much too good to be true. There had to be a glitch, right? My engineering mind had kicked into ultra-high gear, and I couldn't wait to return home to tap every available resource to learn about this seemingly mystical and magical cure.

Another gentleman had joined in listening to the conversation—a man who had selected robotic surgery for his treatment. After a few minutes he jumped into the discussion with both feet and a loose tongue, even in front of several women. He said that he had no love life any longer as a result of his treatment, and that he wishes he had known about proton therapy at the time, but his urologist had not told him about it. He kept trying to close the deal like a used car salesman by asking me repeatedly, "Are you going to do proton?" I thanked him for being honest with me and sharing his insights, but I opined that my knowledge was severely limited to what I had just learned in the past few minutes, so I needed more time to make an evaluation. My reaction caused him to go for the hard sell, and he literally *begged* me to chose proton therapy. He refused to take *no* for an answer. I genuinely appreciated his candor.

These same two proton guys urged me to speak with another gentleman who had remained behind after most everyone left. He, too, had selected robotic surgery some four years earlier. In spite of incredible difficulties that had plagued him since he left the hospital, overall he felt positive about his experience because he was alive. Under the same circumstances, I don't think that I could muster up the same outlook on life that he has. He reported severe urinary issues that began at the hospital following surgery with the application of the catheter, being impotent and having to try many approaches to having some semblance of a love life, and wearing adult diapers requiring multiple changes during the day.

He had written a paper on his experience with robotic surgery, and he provided it to me. Upon reading it, my eyes were really opened as to what this option is really like. He didn't pull any punches, and remember that he felt very positively about it. From that moment on, I knew that I wouldn't permit any surgeon to perform a prostatectomy on me, and especially one using the da Vinci robot. Mentally I severed all ties to my urologist who had recommended what I had now come to realize is a primitive procedure.

Call to me and I will answer you and tell you great and unsearchable things you do not know today.

–JEREMIAH 33:3

Chapter Six

THE AMAZING TRANSFORMATION FROM DESPAIR TO EXPECTATION

WE RACED HOME from the Christmas cancer dinner with a renewed sense of optimism. We knew with absolute certainty that the Holy Spirit had served as the enabler in causing our encounter with the two proton therapy couples.

God's ways are so much wiser and better than our ways. I had been searching feverishly for the right solution to my problem without success. I had hoped and prayed that the obvious answer would manifest itself in a way impossible to miss. I understand why God allowed me to go through this process. He prepared me through all the information gathering over the previous several weeks to arrive at a place where His response would be revealed with absolute clarity. He would answer our prayers, but with His perfect timing. Steel has to be fired as a prerequisite to hardening, and I certainly felt like I had already spent enough time in the flames.

Now I was really pumped up. Was it the time for me to learn His treatment choice for me? Would proton therapy prove to be the answer—*His* answer?

After entering our home, I fired up my laptop and quickly searched for two websites the proton guys had referenced for Florida Proton and Proton Bob. The first was for the University of Florida Proton Therapy Institute (UFPTI) and the second was for Bob Marckini, founder of the Brotherhood of the Balloon. (I'll explain the name later.)

When the Florida Proton site opened, my eyes immediately focused on its mantra, "Hard on cancer, easy on you." I liked the sound of this message, especially after hearing the gloom and doom stories from others who had selected conventional treatment methods. It proved immediately soothing. I literally devoured page after page of information until the website had revealed everything to me that it contained. I clicked over to Proton Bob and went through the same exercise.

What I learned was a real eye-opener. Proton therapy is different. All the *too good to be true* information that the two couples at the Christmas cancer dinner had shared with us was repeated in the two websites. At this stage I thought proton therapy must be the greatest orchestrated sham in medical history or the greatest paradigm shift in treating cancer. However, my optimistic spirit pointed me strongly to believing the latter. I wanted it to be true, but I also recognized that I had to wait for God's confirmation.

Do you know the feeling that occurs when He communicates with you? I've experienced it several occasions during my lifetime, and for me it's different than anything else. I find it impossible to describe to a non-believer whose mind cannot grasp or accept the spiritual truth of a supernatural God who genuinely cares for them. He is the "I AM" who can address any condition and provide comfort, strength, and answers when they are needed most.

On a human level one may experience a hunch, intuition, sense, etc. inside the crevices of his or her mind. However, in these cases, it's only an assumption or feeling based upon a logical analysis arising from past experiences and acquired knowledge.

I've found God's answers to be different. He can respond in many ways, but I'm referring to those occasions when He speaks directly into my mind, heart, and soul—to every single fiber of my being. It's not a voice that I hear with my ears, and He doesn't speak to me through a burning bush or from a cloud. However, He could certainly do so if He wished. After all, He is God.

When He speaks to me, it isn't audible or visible. However–and this is tough to explain–I know absolutely, positively, unequivocally, and with 1,000,000% certainty that it is God communicating to me. It involves no guesswork on my part, no apprehension, no concern, no doubt, no uncertainty, no "ifs, ands or buts".

Cancer is too serious a matter to trust my life to my own limited knowledge and analysis. That's why our prayers were so fervent for God's direction for my treatment method. After all, He is the Great Physician who even knows the number of hairs on my head. His guidance would make it possible to determine the right treatment course, and I just had to wait for His perfect timing to reveal it to me.

On the Monday following the Christmas dinner I contacted Florida Proton and requested an information packet. It arrived the very next day to my surprise and delight. It reconfirmed everything on its website and provided considerable additional information on the treatment, preparation, local housing, etc. Also, it included an application for one to be considered for admission.

I took a deep breath and prayed for God's direction. On Wednesday evening a tremendous feeling of relief swept over me, as I realized that proton therapy was His direction for me.

I filled out the application. On Thursday morning I faxed it to Florida Proton and anxiously awaited its response. Not leaving anything to chance, I also called to make certain that my application had been received.

I was anxious to *get the show on the road.* My urologist had speculated–based upon his hunch and no testing–that my cancer was likely already outside of my prostate and spreading, and that I should make a treatment decision within three weeks. Not waiting for me to make up my mind and assured that I'd accept his recommendation, he took the initiative to tentatively schedule robotic surgery the first week in January. His scare tactic proved ineffective, as divine direction required five weeks for me to know what to do.

Believing that Florida Proton would accept my application and I'd prove with preparatory testing that I'd be a suitable candidate, I contacted my urologist's office and informed it of my decision. It had no response–nothing negative or positive to say. I cancelled the surgery date with confidence and satisfaction. I'd be going to the place about which the urologist had said, "Some guys go to Jacksonville, but it takes two months and who'd want to do that?"

When you hear from God, know that Satan's spiritual attacks will soon follow. Accept his meddling as a blessing, as it will ultimately strengthen your faith as you remain strong and steadfast. God will calm you when Satan tries to disturb you. The experience should increase your resolve to follow His guidance.

On December 23rd Satan launched his attack on me. It first appeared in the form of a telephone call from Florida Proton. A lady from its insurance office informed me that my health insurance company had denied coverage based upon the rationale that proton therapy is experimental, which is sheer nonsense! The first patient was treated in 1954–the same year I entered the first grade; it had cured tens of thousands of people; and, numerous centers existed with many more under development.

When I first learned of my cancer diagnosis, it was shocking. However, I manned up and accepted the reality. When Florida Proton informed me that my health insurance company had rejected my cancer treatment, I literally cried. Over the years my wife and I, like most other people, had diligently paid monthly premiums for our health insurance. One buys it for peace of mind. You hope it's never needed, but it's supposed to be a comfort and help to have it when illness strikes. How the health insurance company could be so callous, so dishonest, and so immoral seemed beyond comprehension.

I quickly learned that the next step was to appeal its rejection. However, this action would take time–time that I didn't have. While waiting on the health insurance company to consider my appeal, my cancer would be spreading. A second rejection would yield further delay. The clock was my enemy.

The very next morning on Christmas Eve, I received a letter from my health insurance company containing the same rejection notice. Satan timed his action perfectly at one of the most joyous times of the year in order to produce the greatest negative impact on my psyche.

However, it didn't provide the effect he attempted to produce. My attitude quickly changed from despondency to resolve. A night of stewing on the injustice that had just happened provided a strong impetus to fight. My being *sad* turned into my being *mad*. A wellspring of confidence flowed through my veins. I knew with absolute certainty that I'd win this battle and beat the health insurance company.

By noon on Christmas Eve I made two phone calls. The first one was to a good friend that I had worked with for many years, who happens to be an attorney specializing in medical malpractice in the same city where the health insurance company is headquartered. Rightly or wrongly, I felt both his reputation and location would be beneficial to my case. The second one was to the lady from the Florida Proton insurance office who had called me the previous day. I informed her that I wished to proceed with the consultation and preparation work in anticipation that I'd be admitted to the program. I also told her about retaining an attorney. My wife graciously agreed that we'd get a second mortgage on our home in order to pay for my treatments. A tentative appointment was scheduled for only three weeks later in mid-January, and I was informed of how much money to bring at the front end.

I am thankful and blessed to have a loving wife who understood why I worked on Christmas Eve and Christmas Day on my insurance appeal. This holiday season would be entirely different from any that we had ever experienced, and certainly not in the usual tradition. As I poured through a massive amount of information on the history of proton therapy, I found more and more to negate any allegation of it being experimental. Every day I compiled a journal on what I had learned and how I felt. It would provide great reference material for the attorneys to find during discovery. By this time I was actually hoping the health insurance company would reject my appeal and my case would proceed to litigation. I had absolute confidence that it'd either approve proton therapy for me or pay through the nose as a result of a court judgment. Either way I'd win, but deep inside, I preferred a litigated settlement that would provide a strong precedent to help others who would fight future battles against them for the same reason.

On the day after Christmas, I received another call from the lady at the Florida Proton office. She suggested that I put my appeal and attorney on hold, and let them handle the first attempt in working with the health insurance company. If they failed, I could take charge of handling it on my own terms. I believed her, accepted her advice, took a deep breath and stepped aside.

Eight days later my wife and I were visiting a favorite shop in the Arts and Crafts Community of Gatlinburg,

Tennessee, and my phone rang. It was the lady from Florida Proton. She informed me that the health insurance company had rolled over, and it would pay for my treatment. This news blew me away, especially since this complete 180-degree reversal had occurred during our nation's major holiday period. I immediately shared the development with my wife, and we could not have been happier. I'm sure the others nearby thought we were perhaps too exuberant in hugging and kissing and high-fiving each other. It didn't matter—we had won!

A couple of hours later we returned home. Our mailbox contained a letter from our health insurance company. It proudly announced that my coverage would pay for proton therapy, and it congratulated me for selecting the world's most cutting-edge technology in curing cancer. It provided some good laughs. A comparison of the two letters, the first with rejection based upon proton therapy being experimental and the second with acceptance based upon it being world-class, proved incredible.

It felt great to kick Satan in the teeth. Now we had the green light to go to Jacksonville.

Trust in the Lord with all your heart and lean not on your own understanding; in all your ways acknowledge him, and he will make your paths straight.

—Proverbs 3:5-6

Chapter Seven

FLORIDA OR BUST

AS A BOY my family would take a vacation to Daytona Beach, Florida, about every three years. I clearly remember my first trip in 1953. It occurred prior to interstate highways on mostly two-lane roads, and the travel time was brutal—about 22 hours from our home in Nashville, Tennessee. We rode in our 1948 Kaiser, a tank of an automobile without air conditioning or much of anything for human comfort. Despite the difficulties of travel in this era, our family regarded it as a tremendous treat. It's humorous now to recall the signs that appeared in the back windows of many cars headed south, which simply stated "Florida or Bust".

On the day that my wife and I drove to Jacksonville to start the process at Florida Proton, it reminded me of the feeling that I had as a kid. I was giddy with excitement—not to see the ocean, but to eliminate my cancer. It's a little strange how age and experience change one's priorities in life.

At this juncture I focused like a laser beam on one goal: gain admittance to the proton therapy program at the University of Florida Proton Therapy Institute (UFPTI). The day after our arrival, we drove to the facility in the heart of the city at the designated appointment time. After signing in with the receptionist, the insurance office marked our first stop. It confirmed our health insurance company had rolled over and accepted its fiscal responsibility to pay for my treatment, and after writing a check for the deductible, I was officially "in"—not "in" the treatment program, but "in" the consultation and preparation phase to determine if my cancer status made me a suitable candidate for proton therapy.

I shuttled a short distance down the hallway to the nurses' station for the staff oncologists. After the customary measurements of my height, weight, body temperature, blood pressure and pulse rate, I was escorted to see the nurse assigned to me—a delightful lady who would shortly know a lot of my personal information, as she took me through an extensive survey on my health status with particular focus on my urinary, bowel, and sexual functions. Although fully clothed, the experience felt like I had been stripped naked. However, I loved it, because I knew this step-by-step and slowly but surely process would make me well and whole again.

A few minutes later the oncologist assigned to me entered the room. Although I would have been grateful for anyone with his specialized knowledge and ability, he turned out to be a perfect match. He possessed a quick wit with a dry sense of humor and exercised considerable patience in answering my exhaustive questions. I suspect many doctors hate having an engineer for a patient. I know that I put mine through the mill in terms of probing him for information and answers. Even without the benefit of going to medical school, as problem solvers engineers assume that they can figure it out. I am no exception.

For the next three days I jockeyed from place to place within the sprawling medical complex of Shands, the teaching hospital for the University of Florida. Some test awaited me at every stop to determine the extent and location of my cancer—a CAT scan, MRI, bone scan, etc. All involved injections of fluids within my veins, turning my arms black and blue from the needle piercings. However, I didn't mind one single bit. It actually thrilled me because I really had to know just how big and bad my cancer was. My urologist back home had speculated (without any testing!) that it was already outside of my prostate, which was the last thing on earth I wanted to hear. With the exhaustive analyses by the pros in Jacksonville, I'd find out for certain.

After running through the gauntlet, I met once again with the oncologist. He performed a digital rectal examination (DRE) to check out my prostate on a touchy-feely basis. He shared the best news that I had received since being diagnosed: all the testing revealed that my cancer was confined and had not spread, and proton therapy would be a suitable treatment to cure me. You can't imagine how happy this news made me. Although I had many weeks of treatments ahead, I already started to sense victory. It gave me great personal satisfaction to have second-guessed my urologist at home and proven him wrong. I smiled like a Cheshire cat that had swallowed the canary. After floating back down to earth, I felt tremendously humbled that God had been and continued to be so gracious to me. I could not thank and praise Him enough.

The fourth day wrapped up my consultation and preparation. A urologist inserted four gold markers carefully in my prostate. They would serve as targeting means for aligning me precisely during the 39 treatments to follow. Next, another CAT scan provided the mathematical model for machining the resin compensators and brass orifices for streaming the proton beam into my body.

The final stop provided a revealing insight into what an actual treatment would be like. Strangely, I had to chug-a-lug a pint of water and wait for a half hour. After stripping down completely except for my socks and donning a revealing hospital gown, I laid on a plastic bladder about four feet long and two and a half feet wide. I had to roll to my side, pull up my leg and raise my knee. A technician lubricated what looked like an arrow with an inflatable balloon in the center of the shaft. He inserted it as far as possible into my rectum and expanded the balloon with a saline solution. I rolled to my back and remained perfectly still on the plastic bladder. X-ray machines rotated in place to provide a three-dimensional view of the gold markers in my prostate. The technician kept jockeying with my position until I met the location criteria. The plastic bladder filled up like foam-in-place packaging, and it formed a body pod that would fit only me. After setting and becoming hard enough, the technician checked my alignment carefully, and a computer controlling the table made minute adjustments in repositioning me perfectly. Once in place, the technician marked crosshairs on each hip corresponding to an X-Y alignment of laser beams shining on me.

During this entire procedure everything was explained clearly and simply. I learned that the prostate moves slightly, and it's important to keep it still during each treatment. This is accomplished by drinking water so that the patient's bladder fills up and nestles the prostate from the top, and by inserting and filling the balloon so that the patient's rectum fills up and captures the prostate from the bottom. This basic procedure, excluding casting the body pod, would be repeated 39 times for every single treatment over eight weeks. Unfortunately, my balloons ruptured on two occasions, so I had to take 41 of them.

Maybe I shared too much information, but now you should have a clear mental picture of the origin of the organization's name for those men who have been treated with proton therapy for prostate cancer, *Brotherhood of the Balloon.*

One's treatment team consists of an oncologist, a physicist, a medical dosimetrist, technician, and nurse. All members play crucial roles in healing a patient. After the consultation and preparation of the past four days, this team executes tasks necessary for administering treatments. Florida Proton sent us back home and scheduled my start date for three weeks later. During this away time for me, they executed the important tasks of identifying the target treatment area, defining the dosimetry plan, machining the compensators and orifices, and reviewing and finalizing the entire treatment program.

We left Jacksonville incredibly happy, thankful, and blessed. On the journey back to East Tennessee, we had much time to reflect on the miracle of what had just occurred. In a few short weeks and if all goes well, my cancer would be a memory never to bother me again. I couldn't wait to get started.

For God did not give us a spirit of timidity,
but a spirit of power, of love and of self-discipline.
–2 TIMOTHY 1:7

Chapter Eight

FAVORED

My wife and I were on a roll—not as a result from our efforts, but in receiving God's favor after weeks of prayer. We witnessed it time and again, as He carved out the jungle of confusion and doubt and showed us His clearly marked path toward health and restoration.

It started with my family doctor's *inability* to resolve my blood pressure issue, which led to the repeated blood work revealing my cancer. It continued with my *failure* to find the right treatment option until His appointed encounter with the two proton therapy couples. The insurance company's *rejection* of paying for my treatment turned 180 degrees after help came my way. My hometown urologist's *mistake* in speculating that the cancer had spread outside of my prostate was corrected by the findings of many days of others' testing. The darkness of his *negativity* became enlightened with the radiance of my oncologist's opinion.

Step-by-step in God's way and timing, my situation changed dramatically with absolute certainty. Inability, failure, rejection, mistake and negativity melted away and were replaced by ability, success, acceptance, correctness, and positivity. The process didn't stop here. It merely picked up the momentum needed to ultimately defeat cancer once and for all.

Finding a place to live temporarily while in Jacksonville became just another hurdle to overcome, albeit minor in comparison to everything else that had occurred. We didn't know anything about the area. The last time we had driven through Jacksonville preceded the existence of its interstate highways. In essence, we knew absolutely nothing.

The house across the street from us had sat empty for months while languishing on the market unsold. Finally someone bought it and our new neighbors moved in. We met them and learned something truly amazing. They had moved to Townsend, Tennessee, from Jacksonville, Florida. Her best friend there was a realtor who handled both sales and rentals. She set us up with this new contact who might be able to help us.

My wife and I are beach people. Florida Proton is located in downtown, and we didn't want to stay nearby. We preferred being close to the beach, and from what we had learned to date, it seemed to us that somewhere on the south side would work perfectly for us. Our neighbor called her realtor friend in Jacksonville who followed-up with us. As it turned out, she lived and worked in Jacksonville Beach and Ponte Vedra, the very area of interest to us. She informed us that her son, who lived in a condominium complex a couple of blocks from the beach, had just moved into town for his job, and he needed to rent his unit. Moreover, he had no issue with our dog joining us—a big hindrance at most other places. We received some photos, and the rest is history. We chose it as our home-away-from-home for our stay in Jacksonville.

Some people may think this whole encounter was simply blind luck—just something coincidental that happened to us. They'd be wrong. I don't believe in luck. However, I firmly believe in answers to prayer. In this case, our *need* for a place to stay was met by a divinely timed encounter.

God's not only great—He's simply *awesome!* In only a month's time, all doubt had yielded to faith; everything bad had changed to good; and, nothing could stop us now!

If you believe, you will receive whatever you ask for in prayer.
—MATTHEW 21:22

Chapter Nine

D-DAY FINALLY ARRIVES

AFTER BEING AT HOME for only a few days, I received *the* phone call that I had eagerly been awaiting. Florida Proton informed me that its preparation work for my treatments would be finished shortly, and that we should come on down.

We packed up all the stuff needed for the next two months along with our dog, and drove 598 miles to the Ponte Vedra condominium so wonderfully made available. The location to the beach, restaurants, the proton center, attractions, and our selected place of worship proved perfect for us. It even met our dog's needs! We felt incredibly blessed to be led to this particular place.

A couple of days later, we drove to the proton center for my first treatment. My spirits were sky-high with feelings of both apprehension and excitement. I had experienced the simulation during the prep work, but now the time had arrived for the *real deal*. I checked in and awaited my appointment time in the lobby. A technician came out and introduced herself, and she instructed me to drink three cups of water immediately and wait for 30 minutes. I gladly obliged, as I could hardly wait to get treatment #1 behind me. The show was finally on the road.

Appropriately later she came out to the lobby to retrieve me. I proceeded to the changing room where I stripped down to my t-shirt and socks and donned a hospital gown. I sat and waited until my turn came up. The check-in at the gantry–the world's most expensive piece of medical equipment, three stories tall and weighing 84 tons–showed extensive quality control measures. As an engineer, the procedure gave me an immediate sense of relief and answered some questions about how one could be ensured of receiving exactly the right treatments without error. After checking in myself on three separate computers, and matching the bar codes on my personal ID, body pod, orifice, and compensator–seven checks–I climbed into my body pod on top of the table for the very first time.

The technicians prepped me using the same procedure as used in the simulation days earlier: balloon insertion, laser alignment, x-rays, and final computer adjustment. I also had to hold a device with both hands and focus intently on not moving a muscle. *My* compensator and *my* orifice were loaded into the proton gun. The technicians gave me final instructions and left the room to initiate the proton delivery.

Of course, they could see and hear me at all times, and even speak to me if necessary. I would have loved being a fly on the wall to hear their conversations inside the control room. I bet they have an incredible variety of stories and jokes about patients that none of us would ever hear.

I lay there totally—well, almost—motionless. I could hear the machine making some slight noises like clicks and whirling, but not much. It's a tense moment, especially at treatment #1. I even hated to see my chest go up and down from breathing, but that wasn't an option. It's inevitable that in this situation, my nose or some other body part would itch, but I'd have to resist the temptation to scratch it. Frank Sinatra music played in the background. The song was *My Way*, which struck me as being quite suitable to my selection of proton therapy as my treatment option.

Delivery of the proton beam isn't immediate, and it isn't determined by the technicians. I learned that both the physicist and oncologist assigned to my case had to give final approval before anything significant would happen. I appreciate the checks and double-checks throughout the procedure that really makes it foolproof.

I know no medical procedure is certain, but the quality control related to proton therapy is as good as it gets.

Without warning the technicians reentered the gantry room to get me out and prepare for the next patient. My time on the table turned out to be only a couple of minutes, but it seemed like an eternity. I asked if the treatment had been performed, and they responded favorably to my surprise.

Wow! I didn't know anything had actually happened. I felt nothing—no penetration of the flesh from billions of protons traveling more than half the speed of light, no heat on my skin or inside my body, no tingling sensation, no pain—just absolutely nothing. "No pain, no gain" popped in my head. However, in the example of proton therapy, this old saying holds no water. It's completely false, and that's to the patient's advantage.

As the technicians brought me down from treatment #1, I asked about the music selection of Frank Sinatra. One told me that from my first impression, they thought it'd be the right choice for me. That cracked me up. I considered myself a young 62, and they viewed me as an old man a generation older than my age. After telling them the types of music that I enjoy, I didn't hear Ol' Blue Eyes' voice again.

Considerable information is readily available that explains proton therapy, how it works, and why it works. I could easily get carried away and dedicate many pages to these subjects. However, that's not my purpose or intent. I'll give you the very short explanation in the simplest language.

Water consists of hydrogen and oxygen. Electrolysis is used to separate them. The hydrogen molecule contains two hydrogen atoms linked by a covalent bond, which is overcome by a high voltage electrical field. The single atom contains only one proton and one electron. Ionization strips the proton away. The positively charged protons must be accelerated to more than one-half the speed of light. This feat is accomplished by a circular accelerator known as a cyclotron. Upon reaching the appropriate speed, the proton beam is sent down a tube and passes through the individualized orifice and compensator and delivered to the patient. The radiation is low at the point of entry and does not harm healthy tissue as it goes into the body to the target location. Through a phenomenon known as the Bragg peak, all the remaining radiation is released precisely at the predetermined delivery point. The radiation effectively destroys the DNA of the cancer cells, which prevents them from reproducing and causes them to die.

I call this the *Homer Simpson* version of what happens. Technical folks would cringe a little bit upon reading it, but that doesn't matter. The main things to appreciate are that proton therapy is proven and it works.

After dressing and returning to the lobby, my smiling wife greeted me. I had a big grin, too! I kept score every single day throughout my 39 treatments. Entering the program, I regarded the score as Cancer-39 and Don-0. Upon completion of treatment #1, I recorded the score as Don-1 and Cancer-38. I had scored, and the game was on. I felt like Secretariat just released from the starting gate, and absolutely no cancer was going to beat me. We celebrated this noteworthy event by dining at a nice restaurant and enjoying the balance of the day.

Your beginnings will seem humble,
so prosperous will your future be.

–Job 8:7

Chapter Ten

JEREMIAH 29:11

AT THE VERY ONSET of my diagnosis, I knew that God would be the healer. Restoration would be for my greatest good and His greatest glory. I had no doubt whatsoever about who was in total control of the situation. I had no doubt whatsoever that He would make me whole. I had no doubt whatsoever that my cancer would be a short-lived blip in my life. These feelings reflected my simple faith in an all-powerful, all-loving, all-knowing, all-wonderful God.

It's an established fact: having a positive attitude promotes healing and increases the likelihood of a successful outcome relative to overcoming an illness. My oncologist's nurse at the proton center shared this simple truth with me and urged me to adopt it wholeheartedly.

She really didn't have to sell me on the idea, because I had bought into it much earlier. I really didn't regard my thought process as reflective of a positive attitude. Instead, I had unwavering faith. I sincerely expected my cancer experience would only reinforce and increase my belief in the Almighty, and that would be a good thing.

Years earlier our younger son left our Kentucky home to attend a Florida college. If you've been in this situation, you can appreciate the apprehension and concern that we had for him. We prayed for him continually. Without fail I sent him a daily e-mail with an uplifting scripture, positive quotation, and personal words of encouragement, and we spoke to him over the phone just about every day. I believed our prayers, my e-mails, and our phone calls would provide a support system that he lacked in a strange town with no family or friends.

I had a similar team that cared for me during my cancer treatments. My wife joined me in Jacksonville for the entire duration of time. She comprised my family support, along with the occasional phone calls and e-mails from our sons and other relatives and friends. The proton center did a fabulous job of getting patients together. We had a fraternity of kindred souls sharing the same treatment experience. I also needed spiritual support, and found it in three places: prayer, church, and Scripture.

It's amazing how adversity makes one more religious. At least that's what happened with me. I admit it's a little shameful and embarrassing, and it doesn't reflect how a real Christian should be. The Bible emphasizes over and over that we are to praise God at all times, even through the ups and downs. Previously when my life moved along smoothly with no bumps or detours, my inclination was to neglect my spiritual growth. However, when troubles arose, and they always did eventually, I would reconnect strongly with God. Don't think too badly of me for this behavior, as it's certain that I have plenty of company who have done likewise. It's just the old sin nature, reflective of our spiritual weakness.

One thing is certain. Going though cancer gave me a great (and needed!) attitude adjustment. It made me mindful of the frailty of life and my absolute dependence upon Him. I never want to let Him down. I never want to stray. Nonetheless, in spite of this knowledge, it'll still happen from time to time, but the great news is that with His unwavering grace, I am always forgiven.

Perhaps it goes without saying that my wife and I prayed feverishly about my healing. She is a real prayer warrior who prays in the biblical way–that is, without ceasing. I can't say enough good things about her level of spiritual support and encouragement, not only through this trying time but always. I know that many others–some unknown–held me in prayer, too, which is really humbling. I'd love the opportunity to express my gratitude to them. Perhaps some day in the next life I'll learn exactly who they were. I surely hope so.

When reading about Jesus in the Bible, it is stunning to realize how much He prayed. If the Son of God placed so much emphasis on communicating with His Father, shouldn't we do the same? I love the stories about how He would sometimes pray out loud so that everyone could hear—not for His benefit, but for them. He set the example, and we would be wise to follow it.

We found a great church, Christ the Redeemer, nearby in Ponte Vedra that provided wonderful music, insightful messages, and friendly people who boosted our spirits. The services could not have been more perfect for someone in my situation.

Most of the music was contemporary in nature with incredible meanings. Songs like *One Thing Remains* by Jesus Culture stuck home so deeply within my heart, and the worship leader featured it almost every week during our time there. If you aren't familiar with it, check it out. The lyrics and accompanying music are amazing:

> *Higher than the mountains that I face*
> *Stronger than the power of the grave*
> *Constant through the trial and the change*
> *One thing... Remains*
> *One thing. . . Remains*

Your love never fails, never gives up
Never runs out on me
Your love never fails, never gives up
Never runs out on me
Your love never fails, never gives up
Never runs out on me

On and on and on and on it goes
It overwhelms and satisfies my soul
And I never, ever, have to be afraid
One thing remains

In death, In life, I'm confident and
covered by the power of Your great love
My debt is paid, there's nothing that can
separate my heart from Your great love...

This song would cause me to tear up and I couldn't help it. What a powerful message that it contains! I'm not a guy who shows much emotion. In fact, in my profession I was called the *Ice Man* for my ability to not let the circumstances get to me when placed in the highest pressure situations. However, that stuff, like being grilled by attorneys in court, was child's play compared to what cancer did to my psyche. It's a disease that can knock anyone down to size, regardless of how *in control* they may feel.

Three different men provided the Sunday messages over the two months of our temporary residency—one special guest from England, and the church's senior and associate pastors. Their words seemed so appropriate for my situation. It's funny how cancer improves one's attention! I heard and comprehended every word. No nodding off from me—I soaked up everything like a sponge. Dr. Daniel Williams, the senior pastor, really helped us. He always had the perfect words to say, whether during the service or to us afterwards. He also did something very meaningful that I don't recall any other pastor ever doing: he prayed specifically for me.

The folks who attended this church proved welcoming, concerned, and positive toward us. Meeting them gave us the wonderful opportunity to witness to them about proton therapy and its ability to cure cancer. Nowadays we return to Jacksonville for my annual checkup, and we always stay a little longer just to visit Christ the Redeemer. Even though it's only once a year, people are still able to call us by name. It's a wonderful feeling to be remembered so thoughtfully.

Scripture provided the third support to us. Its importance cannot be overestimated. After all, the Bible reflects God's will for our lives. Everything we really need to know about life is contained within its pages, dictated by the Holy Spirit and transcribed by men.

You better believe that Bible reading became a key activity for us during this time. Sad to say, it wasn't for me before my biopsy, although to my wife's great credit she had always been diligent about it. So many fascinating passages exist relative to sickness, healing, miracles, faith, encouragement, etc., that one can apply to having cancer.

On that first day of treatment, I decided to find a verse–the perfect verse–to guide me though the next eight weeks. I felt led specifically to Jeremiah 29:11. I particularly like the New International Version (NIV) of this famous passage:

"For I know the plans I have for you," declares the Lord, "plans to prosper you and not to harm you, plans to give you hope and a future."

For me, this verse was it. I believe that it fit me and my situation perfectly. Over and over I heard it in my mind when I thought about the restoration to my body that was taking place.

I decided that it would be beneficial to somehow carry this verse around with me. We stopped in some

Christian bookstores and searched for what they might have. At the second place we stopped, we found a basket of rounded stones with verses written on them. A quick check revealed one with Jeremiah 29:11 based upon the NIV translation. It was perfect! I purchased the stone, and I carried it in my pants pocket every day of treatment as a constant reminder. In fact, I have examined it so many times that the words are barely visible now.

This verse speaks to my heart and soul. It means so much to me that I eventually purchased a stainless steel ring with Jeremiah 29:11 embossed on it. The ring provides an excellent witnessing tool, too—something that I had never considered when I bought it. Sometimes people ask me why I wear two wedding rings or question whether or not my wife and I had repeated our wedding vows, and the conversation opens the door for me to witness to them. Not only did the verse get me through a very tough time in my life, but it has also provided opportunities to tell others about Jesus and what He has done in my life.

When you face a challenge to your health and your life, I encourage you to build a foundation of support. Establish a network with your spouse, children, relatives, friends, and fellow patients. Go for the building blocks of faith that you'll find with prayer, church, and Scripture. Pray without ceasing. Connect with a church. Read the great stories of the Bible, and seize onto a single verse and make it your own Christian mantra.

All of these building blocks of faith make the journey easier. I can't imagine doing it any other way.

"For I know the plans I have for you," declares the Lord, "plans to prosper you and not to harm you, plans to give you hope and a future."

–JEREMIAH 29:11

Chapter Eleven

OFF TO THE RACES

THE NEXT FEW WEEKS moved on methodically with a similar schedule every day. My wife and I would drive the half-hour to the proton center; I'd prep for my treatment by drinking cups of water quickly; a technician would retrieve me from the lobby after a half-hour or so; I'd undress and don a hospital gown, hop on the table, get my balloon, be positioned, shot with protons, lose the balloon, get back into my clothes, and rejoin my wife. From start to finish, excluding the drive time, the whole process would average about an hour or a little more in duration.

As part of this regular routine, I'd meet with my oncologist, his nurse and assistants every single week. They kept close tabs on how I felt and the treatment progress that was being made. One thing about the process, which is for the patient's benefit, is that it's highly personal. In addition to stripping down to the buff and being exposed to young women every treatment, I had to answer a barrage of questions about my bowel movements, urinary outcomes, and sex life. Believe me, I had no difficulty about opening up my life completely, as I felt it important to be extremely forthright in telling them about everything. Knowledge is power, and with more information I felt they could do a better job. However, I recognize that some people–perhaps even the majority–have trouble with these kinds of discussions, fearing embarrassment or not wanting to raise a minor issue. Fortunately, I don't have this encumbrance when talking with medical personnel, which I believe has enabled me to receive the best care possible.

Of course, we participated in the many educational and social functions promoted by the proton center. They served to provide continuous positive reinforcement and encouragement to the cancer patients being treated. Together patients and spouses enjoyed lunches and suppers, informative meetings, field trips to local sites, music and entertainment. We could even sign up for activities like golf, tennis or bridge! It was wonderful! Quite frankly, becoming a social butterfly prevents one from even realizing he or she has cancer. The entire process is really well orchestrated. The proton center treats the whole person. It's not just destroying the cancer cells ability to reproduce and spread. It's also about uplifting one's attitude, knowledge, and spirit.

When not undergoing treatments or participating in scheduled activities, we had considerable down time during our stay in Jacksonville. It's a little embarrassing to share that this cancer treatment has the moniker of *radiation vacation*. It was amusing when people would call to check up on me during our time in Jacksonville. They'd typically ask questions like "do you feel okay?; are you weak?; do you still have your hair?; are you bedridden?; how is the hospital?; have you lost much weight?; etc." I know some of them thought that I really presented a brave front by responding so positively about my situation. I felt great; I enjoyed daily walks; my hair continued growing as always; I only went to bed at night to sleep; all treatments were out-patient; *gaining* weight was a concern; etc.

I kept an ongoing tally of my progress. Day-by-day the protons bombarded the cancer cells and released their deadly radiation. In my mind's eye I could see the battle inside my prostate. I envisioned little cruise missiles flying in and scoring a direct hit on the designated target like a bullseye, exploding and killing the enemy. It was one great battle deserving of a Hollywood movie extravaganza with futuristic weapons and dramatic action! My medical commanders proved overwhelmingly smarter and stronger, and the enemy was annihilated in piecemeal fashion. It could not retreat, because there was no place to go. The perimeter of my prostate had been sealed off, as the first several treatments focused on this region. Then the interior was attacked methodically. Day-by-day, the observers using x-ray equipment could check on the destruction that had taken place. No prisoners were taken. My side didn't even have a POW camp to house them. These cancer terrorists paid dearly for attacking me in a clandestine manner. Their bodies littered the battlefield, dead and unable to recover and regroup.

I know my description is a little silly, but it's how I felt during the treatments. Every few days I'd post an update on my Facebook account. For example, one-third of the way through 39 treatments I showed a tally of *Cancer 26 and Don 13*. I reported the tide had turned just past the halfway mark with *Don 20 and Cancer 19*. I sensed momentum building after two-thirds of the treatments with *Don 26 and Cancer 13*. Finally, I reported complete victory at *Don 39 and Cancer 0*. Of course, my Facebook friends bolstered my spirits with comments recognizing the progress being made throughout the process.

The last week at the proton center provides mixed emotions. On the one hand, it's exciting that the process is almost over and I'd be healed. On the other hand, it's a little sad to be leaving our new friends and temporary Jacksonville home. Our *radiation vacation* would soon be over.

At the weekly proton luncheon and meeting, all the new graduates attending this function for the last time had to stand up and say some words about their experience. Grown men and women stood up and spoke passionately with no embarrassment, alternately crying or laughing. The audience of newbies and continuing patients applauded with every testimony. The mood was absolutely joyous. Can you imagine the positive impact this experience had on the attendees—the people evaluating proton therapy as their treatment option, the newbies who had just arrived, and the patients who still had treatments to go?

Until you experience such an event, it's hard to appreciate just how special it is. Through God and His support team at Florida Proton, my cancer was defeated once and for all. Complete victory is mine to enjoy for the rest of my life.

Think of the analogy of something much more significant than being cured of cancer. Through God's grace by offering Jesus on our behalf, our sin has been defeated once and for all. His complete victory is ours to enjoy for all eternity in heaven.

You restored me to health and let me live.
—Isaiah 38:16b

Chapter Twelve

THE NEW NORMAL

SURVIVING CANCER, regardless of the treatment option that you choose, gives you a new perspective on life. As an initiated member of this club, I can assure you the experience changed me in positive ways.

Of course, deep inside my body, my prostate had been thoroughly radiated by being pounded with protons day-after-day for 39 days. The physical difference resulted in more than a few jokes. Friends and relatives claimed that they could see me glowing in the dark or they smelled bacon cooking, etc. Being the brunt of such goofy jokes came with the territory, and I welcomed such comments as a badge of honor. It's a great feeling to be able to insult cancer.

On the other hand, some folks wanted to keep their distance from me, afraid that my radiation would somehow leak out, contaminate them and give them some horrible affliction. They were sincere, so I held my composure and didn't burst out laughing–at least not directly to their faces. Believe me, it was difficult to hold back.

What happens inside on a cellular level is huge and its importance can't be overemphasized, but you really can't see it, touch it, smell it, hear it or taste it. You accept it through blind faith in believing what your medical team claims along with the proofs that they provide. Only a real skeptic would think otherwise.

I experienced an even bigger change than just killing a few zillion cancer cells. Being presented the key to a new life impacts one profoundly. It affected my psyche like nothing else.

First of all, my spirituality has increased exponentially. I really want to connect with God, to be pleasing to Him, to learn more about Him, and to implement His will for my life. Had my health remained excellent with not a care in the world, I would have missed out on what's truly important in a big way. When you face death or a dramatically life-changing illness, the finiteness of time on this planet comes into clear focus. As the generations preceding you pass away, you realize that you're standing at the front the line, ready to check-out. For a Christian, this realization doesn't cause fear. Rather, it results in anticipation and expectation. You just don't have a firm grasp on what Heaven will be like, but you become anxious with the recognition that you'll soon find out. For this reason, I'm glad that I had cancer!

The drive home from Jacksonville took us through parts of Florida, Georgia, South Carolina, North Carolina, and Tennessee. As we headed north it became more mountainous. We travelled in mid-April, so spring was fully underway. Vegetation had come alive after a winter's dormancy, with trees showing leaves, flowers blooming, and everything growing. Streams fed by rains flowed freely into meandering rivers. Puffy white clouds accented a big blue sky, and the bright sun warmed the earth. Everything around me sparkled with incredible beauty, more so than before. My senses heightened to a much higher level. I saw the little details that I had overlooked previously. For this reason, I'm glad that I had cancer!

My wife and I had been married for decades—38 years at the time of my diagnosis. Her near-death episode seven years earlier had brought us closer together and caused us to make some rather significant life changes. We built a post-and-beam log home in a gorgeous natural area that is as stress-free as any place on earth. I scaled down my employment from working full-time for corporations to working part-time for myself, and I refocused on my wife and our relationship. With me going down a similar road in facing and overcoming a health challenge, I developed a much greater understanding and empathy regarding how my wife feels about life. We now have a common bond achieved from two different directions. The big plus is that our love and appreciation for each other have bloomed to make a more beautiful relationship. For this reason, I'm glad that I had cancer!

Others became much more important to me. A strong desire to contribute and serve hit me. What I do is unimportant, as I try to follow the principles of not letting the left hand know what the right hand is doing, giving in secret, and not seeking the praises of men. Let's just say that my wife and I have a much better understanding now of what it means to love your neighbor more than yourself. The irony is that the one who serves is blessed every bit as much or more than the one who is served. For this reason, I'm glad that I had cancer!

My new normal emerged as being quite different from my old normal. I ditched my cancer and lukewarm Christianity. What radical concepts unfolded in my life: connecting with God, becoming aware of His creation, strengthening my marriage, and serving others. It all sounds downright biblical.

Therefore, if anyone is in Christ, he is a new creation; the old has gone, the new has come!

–2 Corinthians 5:17

Chapter Thirteen

THE BOTTOM LINE: WHAT YOU REALLY MUST KNOW

I AM A CANCER SURVIVOR. I'm going to tell you something that will sound absolutely whacko. If someone had made this statement to me before or at the time of my own cancer diagnosis, I would have thought they were crazy. However, for me, know that it's the absolute truth. *Having cancer proved to be one of the most positive experiences of my life, but only because of proton therapy!*

The best advice that I can give to you is to turn your health over to God. He is the Great Physician. As you personally experience the guidance of the Holy Spirit, you'll see His grace manifested in many ways. Keep the faith! You'll need it through the ordeal you face. The experience will mold you into a much better Christian than before.

My own doctor highly recommended robotic surgery. He opined that if I followed his advice, I'd have a 65% survival probability for ten years, but with quality of life issues that'd make me wish I were dead and a great likelihood of recurrence that would eventually kill me. Doctors, while obviously smart, absolutely don't necessarily know what's right or best for their patients. Think of them as being akin to car mechanics only more educated; at the end of the day they're really just body mechanics. They only give opinions based upon their own limited experience. If your doctor specializes in surgery, he's likely to recommend surgery. If he specializes in radiation, you can be fairly assured that he'll think radiation is your best option. Unfortunately, some in this profession–either consciously or subconsciously–will suggest a procedure that benefits their wallet more than their patient.

At the end of the day, you are responsible for your own health. It's not up to your doctor or your spouse or your other relatives or friends. Look in a mirror–you are the decision-maker; you and no one else. You must live with the consequences of your own decision.

Fortunately, I learned about proton therapy via a God-appointed meeting with two new (and dear) friends, and it literally changed my life. It's important to tell others about this world-class, cutting-edge technology, because even now most people learn about it through word-of-mouth. As a direct beneficiary I have an ethical responsibility to spread the good news.

I don't want to paint too rosy a picture and one that may be unrealistic for your situation. Proton therapy isn't for everyone. While it's suitable for curing many cancers, it isn't a cure for all types. Some cancers that would normally be treatable may be too advanced for it. Not everyone can afford it or take the time required for treatments. (However, you'll learn in the next chapter that tremendous progress is being made in addressing these issues!) Regardless of one's situation, proton therapy is absolutely worth checking out. Do not hesitate to talk with the experts at a proton center who work with it day-in and day-out. It just might be the right solution for you. I pray that it is, and that you will benefit as I have.

Your health insurance company will likely reject proton therapy as a treatment option, claiming it's experimental or some other nonsense. Don't take the rejection lying down. You can beat them, and your proton center may assist you. Your insurer is simply taking the easy way out to reduce its out-of-pocket costs. It doesn't care about your continuing quality of life. They want you to choose the lowest priced option. Many people—and this makes me sad and disappointed—simply roll over and don't challenge the decision. I'm talking about your life. Don't let some office clerk at your health insurance company determine what you can and can't do to preserve it.

Proton therapy treatments take some time. My course required almost nine weeks. Many people may not have the opportunity for this option unless they live near one of the few proton centers that exist or can make special arrangements relative to their employment in order to go out-of-town. Believe me: it's worth the price even if tremendous sacrifices must be made. However, only you can determine what you're willing and able to give up to do it.

Proton therapy possesses incredible advantages over conventional treatment options. First, it requires no surgery and it's done on an out-patient basis. Think about it: no banking of blood or transfusions, no anesthesia, no incisions, no cutting out tissue, no stitches, no pain upon awakening, no tubes attached to your body for days, no overnight stays at a hospital–just nothing! You have a lot of free time to either work or enjoy a *radiation vacation* when eliminating your cancer.

Second, there is no recovery time. After my last treatment, we joined our fellow patients and spouses for a victory meal, packed up our automobile and drove 598 miles back home. The next day we hiked a robust 3-1/2 miles in the Great Smoky Mountains National Park. The following week we played golf three times while walking the course. If I had followed my first doctor's advice, after one week I'd still be bedridden, depending upon my wife to help me, and looking forward to going to the bathroom on my own.

Third, I had no *permanent* side effects. I emphasize the word *permanent,* because I experienced some side effects during and after treatments. However, and this is important, they were minor, manageable, and temporary. It was no biggie whatsoever–more of a little irritant than anything else. Importantly, the proton center has remained in frequent and regular contact with me to ensure that I don't have any issues, and I can reach a medical expert there at any time should I need them for any reason.

Fourth, I have no quality of life issues! This one is a real biggie, and in my opinion, just as important as the fifth advantage listed next. Remember my original *cut and collect* doctor told me of permanent changes that would make me wish I were dead. I'm absolutely delighted to report that as a direct result of the phenomenal precision of proton therapy, I don't wear diapers and I have a love life–two outcomes that surgery couldn't deliver in my case.

Fifth, my cancer is gone. The proton therapy destroyed the cancer cells' DNA and their ability to divide, grow, and spread. While surgery would have likely assured my eventual demise from prostate cancer, I chose the path less travelled, and now my survival probability is 99.5%. I really like my current odds a lot better. Few things in life, particularly in the area of one's health, carry such a high confidence level.

If you have been diagnosed with cancer and are considering your treatment options, I implore you to compare proton therapy against anything else. In my opinion, it's unmatched and there's nothing else anywhere close *if you're a candidate for it*. Very honestly and sincerely, I tell you that I do not feel like I have ever had cancer.

I've reported my own experience in beating cancer. Be mindful that I am not a doctor and I offer no medical advice to your specific situation. What I have written about myself may not apply to you. Everyone is different. However, my experience is pretty typical of what other proton patients have also reported to me. My sole purpose is to educate you about another cancer treatment option that you likely don't know. When you make your own analysis, I encourage comparison of proton therapy to any other treatment option.

In the whole scheme of living, the best decisions I have ever made in my life are acceptance of God's grace as number one, marrying my spouse as number two, and proton therapy as number three. They have been radically life-changing and have continued to bless me tremendously today. You cannot imagine how much these decisions and the outcomes that have resulted from choosing them have meant to me.

I am cancer-free and absolutely convinced that prostate cancer will never harm me again. I know that the victory is not only over an insidious disease, but a sound defeat of Satan, too. God's love and care, as exemplified by everything that happened to me, using the vehicle of proton therapy and its skilled medical professionals, made it happen.

These kinds of experiences deepen one's faith and genuinely add to one's life in ways that are truly important. As I wrote previously, my wife dodged death from a widow(er)-maker heart attack that would have killed the vast majority of people, but she survived only because of God's goodness to her (and to me!) What we have overcome as a couple in our individual health challenges has yielded a harvest of tremendous blessings for our ultimate benefit. Both of us are glad to have experienced Satan's attacks and death threats on our lives. They have made us better Christians, more cognizant of how much God truly cares for us, and firmly focused on what is really important in life.

Having cancer proved to be one of the most positive experiences of my life, but only because of proton therapy! I pray it does the same for you.

For it is by grace you have been saved, through faith—and this is not from yourselves, it is the gift of God—not by works, so that no one can boast.

—Ephesians 2:8

Chapter Fourteen

THE NEW PARADIGM FOR CURING CANCER

As you've obviously noted by now, I'm a huge fan of proton therapy. After all, not only did it save my life, but it preserved it as well.

The obvious question one might ask is, "If proton therapy is so great, why isn't it offered everywhere?" The answer won't surprise you: it's all about *money*, pure and simple.

One proton gantry with supporting hardware like a cyclotron is the most expensive piece of medical equipment in the world. A typical proton center has three gantries, but the capital expense to build one includes so much more. The facility to house one has concrete and steel walls typically around ten feet thick, and the support infrastructure for things like enormous electricity and water supplies cost enough to choke a horse. Everything lumped together carries a price tag that ranges from $120 to $200 million for one proton center.

For this amount of money, several (but not all) cancers can be cured. By comparison, a well-equipped hospital may run $70 to $120 million, and it is capable of addressing many diseases and not just cancer. At the end of the day it's safe to say that a proton center requires a monetary investment of roughly 2X that for a regular hospital. It's a huge disparity.

I went to the University of Florida Proton Therapy Institute in Jacksonville. It was the fifth center built in the United States. At the time of my treatment, there were a grand total of nine proton centers in the country.

Today the situation is quite different. More and more centers are popping up. Near my home in Knoxville, Provision Center for Proton Therapy became number fourteen in January 2014. At this writing many others are under some phase of development ranging from seeking financing to actual construction.

Unless some brainiac comes up with something better and cheaper, like a piece of candy that stops cancer cells dead in their tracks, I believe proton therapy will be the cancer treatment choice of the future. Today's conventional methods will seem antiquated and ineffective by comparison.

Of course, the cost of a single proton center translates to a high treatment cost for each patient. In turn, insurance companies balk at paying for it. The situation is a classic chicken-and-egg problem.

As a clear example, most people realize that when a person is diagnosed with pancreatic cancer, it's a virtual death sentence. The one treatment option that gives someone a chance of surviving if the diagnosis is made early: proton therapy. However, some insurance companies employ a *delay to death* strategy—that is, they disapprove the treatment and cause the patient to go through an appeal process that may be lengthy enough for the patient to die before the insurance company has to pay. It stinks and it's immoral, but it's reality.

The real key for proton therapy acceptance is lowering the price of treatment and passing the savings on to patients. The really great news is that such a change is fast becoming a reality.

First, a new protocol known as hypo-fractionation permits qualified candidates to receive a higher radiation dose with fewer treatments. The price compares favorably with conventional Intensity-Modulated Radiation Therapy (IMRT). As a result, it'd be totally illogical for an insurance company to reject coverage for a patient who selects proton therapy over a conventional method. This protocol also benefits the patient by reducing the timeframe by half.

Second, imagine the positive impact of new generation proton therapy equipment being invented that could be manufactured at a much lower cost than existing equipment and be installed in a conventional facility. Such an outcome would reflect a true *paradigm shift*–that is, a fundamental change in approach or underlying assumptions.

This idea sounds nice but perhaps a little too good to be true. However, it's actually happening in East Tennessee. Provision Health, the parent corporation for the Provision Center for Proton Therapy, also has an engineering and manufacturing subsidiary called ProNova. It is creating the next generation proton therapy equipment that will transform the way some cancers can be cured. Prices will drop as progressive hospitals will start adding this capability in 2016.

Both developments, hypo-fractionation and lower-cost equipment, represent huge steps in crashing the barriers that have hindered this phenomenal technology from spreading. My hope and expectation are that proton therapy as a cancer treatment option will spread like wildfire across our country and bring its life-saving and life-preserving healing to millions.

We should never lose sight of an important point. None of this progress would or could be made without God. All good and perfect gifts come from Him—even proton therapy.

Through him all things were made; without him nothing was made that has been made."

−JOHN 1:3

CLOSING

My desire is that this simple book has enlightened you. Hopefully you've learned something new, and maybe you've selected proton therapy as your cancer treatment option. Regardless of what decision you make relative to your own battle, I urge you to keep the Great Physician as your primary focus. My prayer is that you, too, will survive and thrive in beating cancer.

ACKNOWLEDGEMENTS

Writing a book isn't a solitary exercise. This one is no exception, as my family and friends contributed their encouragement, talent, and time to make it happen. I give them my heartfelt appreciation for helping me.

I thank Allen Jackson, who motivated me to find the Holy Spirit's direction for my life, which inspired me to write this book. He provided a wonderful endorsement of the work as well.

My sons, Brian and Andrew Denton, reviewed my writing with a close eye, and they made excellent recommendations for improving my original draft. They also wrote the Foreword. Andrew's wife, Ashlee, gave her creative talent for the photograph on the cover.

Sulynne (aka Susie), my wife and love of my life, kept after me to continue writing on those days that I didn't feel like doing so. As a witness and confidant to my entire experience of beating cancer, she served as the fact-checker to the accuracy of the story.

Dr. Terry Douglass and Dr. Nancy Mendenhall, two giants in the proton therapy world, did far more than I expected with their insightful critiques of my writing. I'm humbled by their contributions to my story. You won't find two more dedicated people focused on eradicating cancer.

Two spiritual mentors, Dr. Daniel Williams and J. P. Wilson, taught me so much about being a Christ-follower. I treasure their friendship. Both graciously read my book and wrote supportive reviews.

Phillip Jackson shared his valuable insights into the world of publishing, and he directed me to the right people at the right time to put my story in print. Gwyn Kennedy Snider of GKS Creative transformed my work into the beautiful result you see in this book.

I acknowledge all the unnamed folks who had confidence in me, and always expressed the right words to keep me focused. Lastly, I applaud the many people who told me their own personal stories of battling cancer.

CALMING THE STORM

_____

_____

_____

_____

_____

_____

_____

_____

_____

_____

_____

_____

_____

_____

_____

_____

_____

_____

_____

_____

_____

_____

_____

_____

_____

.